The ABC's to Health and Healing

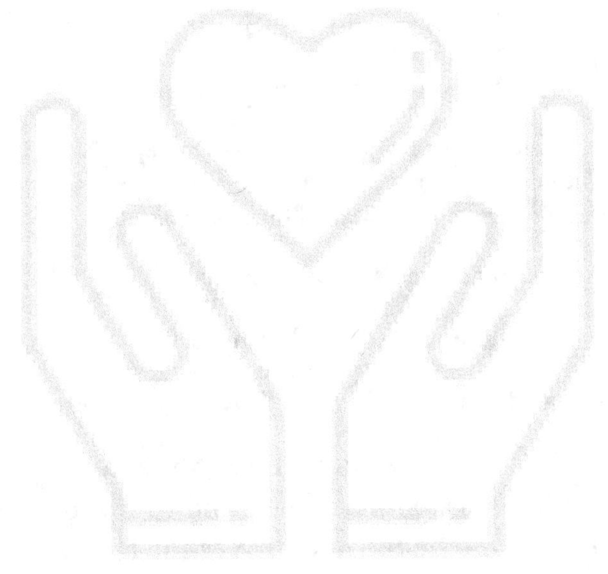

Dr. Chad Costantino

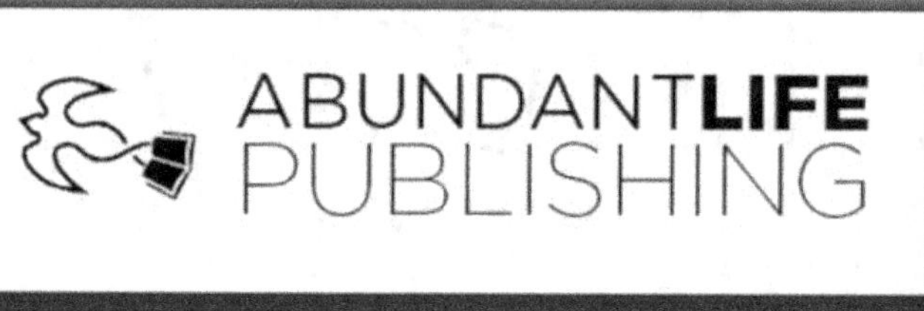

Edited by: Gavriela Powers

Assistant Editor: John Hall

Cover and Interior Design: Gavriela Powers

We hope you enjoy this book from Abundant Life Publishing. Our goal is to help you and your little ones live, laugh, and be the light of Yeshua (Jesus)!

Abundant Life Publishing

Salisbury, NC

Printed in the United States of America

Contents

Dedication

 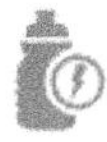 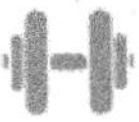   

This booklet will be given for free to as many Veterans as we can possibly reach; we dedicate this booklet to every Veteran out there, whose sacrifices, for us, have a lot to teach.

The Effects of War on Soldiers

By Eavan Costantino

War has been a part of human history for centuries; in all circumstances, it has not only taken the lives of countless soldiers, but it has inflicted the other effects that can change a perons's life forever.

Many soldiers come back home from war with mental trauma, physical injuries, and other negative marks that the horrors of war inflict upon them. It is not only moral, but also logical for the government to use more of the tax payer's money to fund programs that make an effort to help veterans who face issues caused by their experiences of war.

The most common physioclogical issues found in veterans are depression and PTSD. Sometimes these psychological issues occur because the brain attempts to deal with trauma and fails to do so. PTSD was discovered when people noticed symptoms in Vietnam veterans. It was not defined as a specific disorder until the 1980s. When interviewed in an NPR report, President Richard Nixon's drug czar stated that approximately 40% enlisted soldiers in the Vietnam war had tried heroin, and that half of those men had become addicted to the drug.

According to American Military doctors, the number of suicides in the Army rose by 80% after the war with Iraq began, and as of about 2010, about 22 veterans commit suicide daily. A survey by the IAVA discovered that 17% of Iraq and Afganistan veterans are jobless as of January 2012. They also found out that 67% of these veterans do not think that the mental healthcare being offered to them is adequate.

Research has also discovered that veterans in the present time are at a higher risk for mental health problems such as PTSD, suicide, depression, and substance abuse. Another study shows that 30% of soldiers develop mental problems within three to four months of being home from war. These numbers are more than likely rising, since this information was found several years ago.

As of recently, Canada has deployed over 27,000 troops to Afganistan. In February of 2010, the Canadainn Forces said that 529 soldiers have been physically injured in action from 2002 to 2009. Nine-hundred-and-thirteen other soldiers have experienced "non-combat injuries". Pierre Daigle (a member of the Candian Forces) said that

17% of the 27,000 troops that have been deployed are expected to show mental health problems. Since 2007, personell who have suffered physical injuries during combat have been able to remain in military service indefinitely. Sadly, some soldiers with physical limitations have been declined opportunities for promotion.

More research has also proven that approximately 20% of Iraq and Afganistan veterans began drinking, or doing drugs when they returned to the United States. About 55% of women and 38% of men have admitted to being victims of sexual harassment during military service, and between 10-20% of Iraq and Afganistan veterans have suffered from a traumatic brain injury. Nearly 11-20% of veterans who gone to war in Iraq or Afganistan have been diagnosed with PTSD.

While all of these effects may give a sense of hopelessness to a suffering veteran, there are organizations in the United States that make an effort to provide services to help them. For example, one of these helpful groups is Homes for our Troops. They spend 89% of their donations on aiding veterans. Only 5% of their donation money is spent on fundraising.

Another organization that has made a noticeable impact when helping veterans is the Wounded Warrior Project. Their mission is to provide assistance to military personnel who have been injured after 9/11. They have received $312 million dollars in donations, and they used 60% of that money for the aid of wounded veterans. Roughly 34% of the money donated to them is used for fundraising.

While these organizations are extremely beneficial for veterans, there are still ways that an average American citizen can help. One can sponsor a companion dog for a veteran suffering from Post Trauamtic Stress Disorder with the help of an organization called Puppies Behind

Bars. This group lets inmates in several prisons train dogs to help veterans who have need of one. One can also send a care package, or a letter, to a veteran through Operation Gratitude. Simply saying "Thank you" to a veteran can also impact them, because it shows them that they are respected for their service to America.

After studying the effects that war can inflict on soldiers, it would only make sense to believe that providing more care for veterans that are suffering is something that the American government should make a high priority. This would only begin to pay them the respect and gratitude that they deserve from Americans as a whole. Therefore, it is a logical and moral obligation for the government to put the money of a taxpayer to good use by funding programs that help soldiers and returning veterans with the traumatizing injuries inflicted on them by the horrors of war.

Introduction

 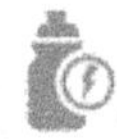 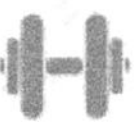   

We would like to introduce to you Abundant Life Publishing's new line of ABCs booklets! In these booklets we use rhyming to help your memory retain what you read; we will also assign each letter of the alphabet with a word that you will need! We will explain how this word relates to the topic of the booklet, in this case, *health and healing*, as we go along. By the end of each booklet, we hope your spirit will feel sturdy and strong!

<u>A</u>bba Father

<u>B</u>eloved Yeshua (Jesus Christ)

<u>C</u>ounselor the Holy Ghost

<u>S</u>pirit Guide!

It is obvious that Abba wants us to recognize our beloved Kingdom Identity and speak His promises over you and me! We must line up our thoughts with His Word, if we are to prosper and endure. Whose voice are we following, and how can we be sure? Being Kingdom Minded is the cure!

In this booklet, we will be discussing the process of health and healing from a non-medical point-of-view. This booklet teaches principles about health and healing from a spiritual perspective, which can and will, in turn, affect your physical outcome over time. This booklet is not meant to substitute the advice of any medical professionals in cases of serious life-threatening illnesses or emergency situations. Always consult your healthcare professional before beginning a new health supplement of any kind, and always endeavor to know your own body before trying to push your limits physically.

A — Anointing

  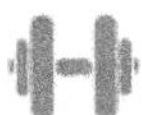 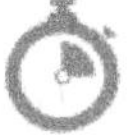  

The Bible contains so many rich principles that teach us how to achieve health and healing every day; bringing the sick among you to the elders of the congregation and having them prayed for and anointed is one way!

An anointing represents the complete smothering and outpouring of the Holy Spirit into the human soul; symbolically speaking, when you receive an anointing from an elder believer, God makes you inside, a little more whole. An anointing is meant to cover every aspect of your being; to help you hear better, walk better, and see more clearly.

Sickness can often be a sign of sin in someone's life, although that is not always the immediate case. The Scripture in the Bible that teaches to pray and anoint over sick people also says their sins will be forgiven and they will be given grace.

One important step to health and healing is making sure that you are anointed by the Holy Spirit regularly; this will help you to stay healthy and always clearly see! One hindrance to health and healing is often a lack of anointing; a lack of the Holy Spirit Who is the One Who is appointing. Guard your health and healing today and ask God for a supernatural anointing to be sent your way!

Check Point

When was the last time you were prayed for and anointed by an elder of a believing congregation? What was your experience? When was the last time you personally asked God to send His Holy Spirit to anoint you? Endeavor to ask God every day for a fresh anointing!

Exclamation Point   !

"Is any sick among you? let him call for the elders of the church; and let them pray over him, anointing him with oil in the name of the Lord: And the prayer of faith shall save the sick, and the Lord shall raise him up; and if he has committed sins, they shall be forgiven him."

- James 5:14-15

"All healing is essentially a release from fear." - Anonymous

Bonus Word   

A can also be for *Alkaline*; did you know that cancer cannot exist in an alkaline environment? Drinking plenty of alkaline water can add to your daily health and healing!

B — Balanced Diet

 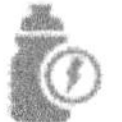 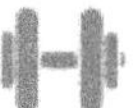 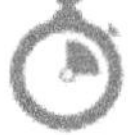  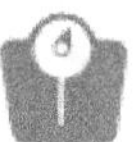

A balanced diet can be hard for some to achieve, especially if you're used to eating whatever you want whenever you want. If you don't keep a balanced diet in mind over the years, it will eventually come back to haunt!

Achieving a balanced diet also means being in tune with what your body needs; some people are lower on iron, while others have higher protein needs. You can learn all about the diet your body needs by going to a nutritionist; they test your blood levels and a few other things to help you find the diet that is best!

Achieving a balanced diet also means killing the unhealthy cravings you have trained your body to feel; abstaining from junk food and processed foods can make a change overnight, for real!

Your mind also needs a balanced diet; quiet times, reflective times, active times, singing times, times of hard work and times of relaxation. If your mind is not on a balanced diet, it will shake loose your entire body's foundation!

Check Point

What is the biggest struggle you have with keeping a balanced diet? Write down three goals you have for your mind and body in achieving a better diet, then pray and ask God to help you stay accountable to achieving those goals!

Exclamation Point

!

"But he answered and said, 'It is written, Man shall not live by bread alone, but by every word that proceedeth out of the mouth of God." - Matthew 4:4

Bonus Word

B can also be for *Blood*; did you know that the Bible says the life is in the blood (Leviticus 17:11)? If our blood isn't healthy, the rest of our body will suffer, too. If we eat too much fat, our blood will become too thick and our arteries clogged!

C – Crying

Science has shown that there are three different kinds of tears: basal, reflex, and psychic. Each kind of tear has its own purpose and its own kick. Basal tears are there all the time, keeping the eye moist and protected. Reflex tears are the kind that are produced when your eye gets onion juice in it or other foreign entities are detected.

Psychic tears are the kind that are produced when you need to have an emotional cry; beneath a microscope, those kinds of tears look completely different than the others, and here's why: emotional tears release toxins from within our bodies that need to be gotten out. When we cry emotional tears, we are actually doing something that is healthy for us, without a doubt!

Crying is a healthy action that needs to be nurtured and not held back; crying when you feel like you need to can lead to a healing process that you may have previously lacked. Crying does not show weakness or mean that you're not strong enough to carry on; crying shows that you are intelligent and doing what God created your body to do all along!

Check Point

When was the last time you had a healthy cry? Do you cry often, or are you afraid to cry? Why or why not? What kind of thoughts do you need to change to have a healthier perspective on crying?

Exclamation Point

!

"They who sow in tears shall reap in joy." - Psalm 126:5

"Instead of saying, 'I'm damaged, I'm broken', say, 'I'm healing, I'm rediscovering myself, I'm starting over.'" – Anonymous

Bonus Word 

C can also be for *Chemicals*; today, chemicals are added into just about everything. Our clothing, our food, our hygiene and beauty products. Eliminating as many chemicals from your daily life as possible will greatly increase your health and healing, and that of your family's, too!

D - Diligence

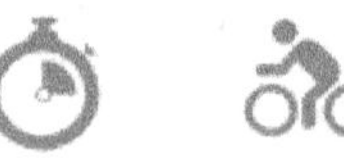

In the journey to health and healing, diligence is needed in measures that abound. Maintaining health and healing daily is something that cannot be done without diligence all around! Health and healing are things that are progressive, and need maintenance and adjustments every day; diligently keeping an eye on what you eat, think, and say!

Having diligence in your health means knowing when you need to push your boundaries and when you need to respect them; having diligence in your health means following a diet plan and not just eating or doing whatever you want on a whim.

Health and healing as a lifestyle, especially after you have gotten sick and need a new beginning, means being willing to start from scratch, learn new things, and really go for the winning! Having diligence in your relationship with God is absolutely essential to having health and healing every day; without diligence in seeking Him first, sickness and death will have their way.

Check Point 

Do you get discouraged with your health and healing at times? What causes that discouragement? List three ways you desire to be more diligent in your health and healing, and then pray and ask God to hold you accountable to achieving those goals!

Exclamation Point 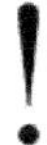

"A man shall be satisfied with good by the fruit of his mouth: and the recompense of a man's hands shall be rendered unto him."- Proverbs 12:14

Bonus Word

D can also be for *Detox*; flushing out your system from time to time with a juice fast or a water detox is essential to resetting your organs and beginning anew in your journey to health and healing. Detoxing your mind is also essential to your health; the more junk that compiles in your mind, the more it will pollute your body. Detox today with prayer, fasting, and praise and worship!

E – Essential Oils

Essential oils are one of nature's best kept secrets to health and healing. Essential oils can enhance, in some cases, instantly, how you are feeling! Essential oils have a unique compound that enhances the good bacteria in your body and attacks the bad; there is an essential oil out there for any symptom of sickness you have ever had!

Essential oils are used by holistic doctors who prefer natural remedies over pharmaceutical medicines; essential oils are organic and natural, so you can use them time and time again! Each essential oil has a unique purpose and should be researched thoroughly and with care before use; if you don't know what you're doing when it comes to essential oils, you may want to call a truce!

The essential oil market can be tricky, but once you've found a brand and company that you can trust, your body and mind will realize essential oils are an absolute must! They work in harmony with your body without causing harmful side effects; not using them sooner has been my only regret!

<u>Essential Oils for Anxiety:</u>

Lavender, Yling Yling, Rose, Vetiver, Chamomile, Bergamot.

<u>Essential Oils for Gut Health:</u>

Ginger, Peppermint, Clove, Thyme, Fennel, Tarragon, Tea Tree, Oregano.

<u>Essential Oils for Brain Health:</u>

Lemon, Vetiver, Lavender, Frankincense.

Essential Oils can be diffused, ingested, or massaged on to skin with a carrier oil such as coconut oil or olive oil.

Check Point

Have you ever used Essential Oils? Why or why not? What kinds of symptoms do you have that you would like to find an oil to help with? Write them down and then do some research!

Exclamation Point

!

"Oil for the light, spices for anointing oil, and for sweet incense…" - Exodus 25:6

"When 'I' is replaced with 'we', even 'illness' can become 'wellness'." – Anonymous

Bonus Word

E can also be for *Exercise*; exercising the mind and body regularly is absolutely essential to maintaining your

health and healing. Without proper exercise, muscles begin to lose their memory and your mind can also become complacent. Exercising your body can mean taking a daily walk, and exercising your mind can mean endeavoring to learn one new thing a day.

F - Faith

 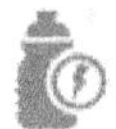 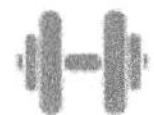 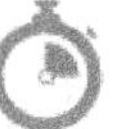  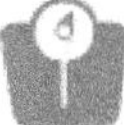

Faith is the key element in any health and healing process. The Bible tells us that without faith, it is impossible to please God (Hebrews 11:6), so He expects our faith and nothing less! Faith is a disease-killer, a sickness killer, and a healer of both body and mind. Faith is one of the best medicines that you will ever find!

That's because faith is our Kingdom Currency, the stuff of the heavens that we spend and save like money here on earth. Faith gives us value and enhances our heavenly worth. Faith gives us access to miracles and healing divine; through faith we are saved, and by faith we shine!

Sometimes, even someone of great faith can fall ill, and there are a number of reasons that may occur. If we don't take proper care of our bodies, over time this can happen, or even your genetics may infer. Sickness can sometimes come from sin or can also sometimes be an attack; sometimes God can use sickness as a way to get our attention back.

Whatever the reason for illness may be, in the end, faith is still a cure. In the very least, faith will guard your heart and mind even when your body isn't sure. Faith opens up doorways of blessings and healings galore; if it's anything we need, it's a lot of faith, even more!

Check Point

When was the last time your faith was tested through an illness or disease? What was your experience? List three things you would like to have more faith about in your process of health and healing.

Exclamation Point   !

"You will keep him in perfect peace, whose mind is stayed on You, because he trusts in You."

— Isaiah 26:3

"Healing most times needs an atmosphere of faith." – Benny Hinn

Bonus Word 

F can also be for *Fasting*; fasting has numerous benefits for your health. It can help reset your gut balance, detoxify your liver and kidneys, and promote healthy cell regeneration. Fasting for three days at a time regularly can help you maintain a great balance for your health and healing. There are many types of fasting, so you should research which one is best for you.

G – Guesswork

 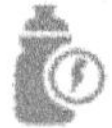 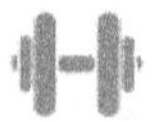  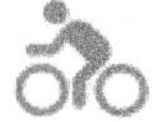 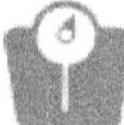

Sometimes doctors are put into medical situations they weren't prepared for in school; in these times they rely on their education and more research to identify the problems and what are the right tools. In these times, they make educated guesses in which direction to start; they look at symptoms, the healthy history of the patient, and major organs like the heart.

In moments like these, when believers are faced with a health situation that not even the doctors know, the guesswork can be eliminated by relying on the Holy Spirit, and letting His wisdom flow.

There once was a time when doctors knew that in order to heal a person completely, they needed mind, body, and soul to have attention. Nowadays doctors rarely address the soul of a person, and certainly not the spirit to mention!

When it comes to health and healing, the guesswork can always be eliminated by seeking God and His answers first. Forgetting to put Him at the top of your go-to list for healing will just make things worse!

Check Point 

When was the last time you asked the Holy Spirit to reveal wisdom to you about a reason you were sick, or how to properly heal yourself? On your journey to health and healing, make sure to put the Holy Spirit at the top of your go-to list for consultation!

Exclamation Point   !

"But seek first the kingdom of God and His righteousness, and all these things shall be added to you."
– Matthew 6:33

"What you are living is the evidence of what you are thinking and feeling, every single time." – Abraham Hicks

Bonus Word   

G can also be for *Gut Health*; gut health is more important than most people realize. The health of your stomach can determine the health of the rest of your body. To maintain good gut health, it's important to be sensitive to what gives you good and bad digestion when you consume food.

H – Heaven

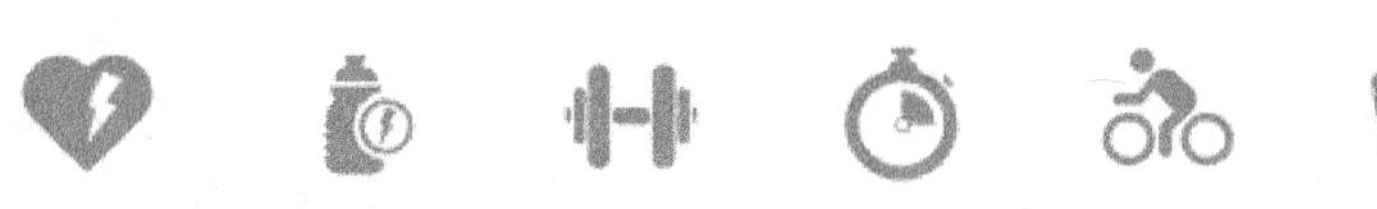

Yeshua (Jesus) taught us to pray in Matthew 5 for God's will to be done on earth as it is the heavens, and this is an important aspect to health and healing. That's because there is no sickness in the heavens, and when we pray that way, it leaves the powers of darkness reeling!

In our journey to health and healing, it's proper to maintain a heavenly state of mind; keeping your thoughts set on things above so that your thoughts produce emotions of the heavenliest kind! Our emotional health is as important to our bodily health, because our emotions affect the way our body functions; when we realize this, we truly come to an important junction.

The principles of heaven are directly applicable to our everyday lives for health and healing as a lifestyle. Serving God by serving others, reading His Word, singing

Him praises, having faith in scary situations, not only protects you, but makes your time here on earth more worthwhile!

Check Point

How often do you check your mind to see if it is aligned with the heavens? How do you think this affects your everyday health and healing? What are three adjustments you would like to make to ensure that your mind, body, and soul are operating in the principles of heaven?

Exclamation Point !

"But if the Spirit of Him who raised Jesus from the dead dwells in you, He who raised Christ from the dead will also give life to your mortal bodies through His Spirit who dwells in you." – Romans 8:11

"I believe the greatest gift you can give to your family and to the world is a healthy you." – Joyce Meyer

Bonus Word 

H can also be for *Holistic*; holistic medicine is an "alternative medicine" because it is an alternative to pharmaceuticals. God created everything we need to derive from the earth for our health and healing; holistic medicine is an all-around better approach to medicine because it uses only natural properties.

1 — Internal Affairs

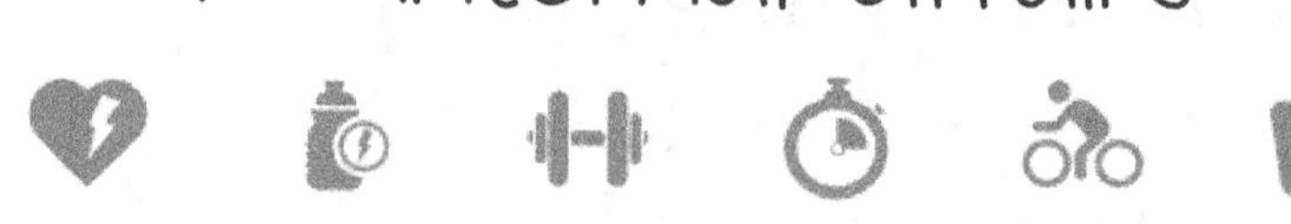

Today's pop culture focuses a lot on the outside of a person, rather than what's inside; pop culture has it backwards, because the internal affairs are always the beginning of what manifests on the outside.

Your internal affairs are the issues of your heart; what do you keep your thoughts focused on, and what in your faith sets you apart? Your internal affairs are essential on your journey to health and healing; thinking bad thoughts constantly will leave your body badly feeling!

Sicknesses always begin on the inside, and the outside just catches up after the sickness has grown roots; in health and healing it's essential that you investigate every open door, and what the enemy desires to loot! Remember that he doesn't come to steal away your material things; he desires to plant seeds of doubt and anger, the pains that really sting!

You can reprogram your mind by doing daily practices of examining your thoughts and redirecting them as needed; that way, you'll find immediately whatever the enemy seeded!

Check Point

How often do you take inventory of your thoughts? What are some changes you would like to make to examine your thoughts more consistently? How much do you believe that your thoughts affect the way you physically feel?

Exclamation Point   !

"Therefore, whether you eat or drink, or whatever you do, do all to the glory of God." – 1 Corinthians 10:31

"Finding lack in others is not the path to liking what you see in yourself." – Abraham Hicks

Bonus Word 

I can also be for *Intimacy*; having intimacy with the Holy Spirit will be the best safeguard for your health and healing journey available. That's because it's part of the Holy Spirit's job to guard you, reveal things to you, give you wisdom, and protect your Temple, because that is where He dwells!

J - Jealousy

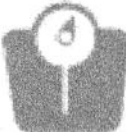

The Bible literally teaches that jealousy is as rottenness to the bones (Proverbs 14:30). That means, under the influence of jealousy, your health and healing eventually turn into stones! Eliminating jealousy from your thoughts and mind is essential on your journey of health and healing; your body won't be healthy if your mind is toxic and your peace, your thoughts are stealing!

It suffices to say that your overall health and healing in body also depends a lot on the condition of your mind; if you are diligent in eliminating toxic mindsets, health and healing you'll readily find!

Jealousy takes your focus off of your blessings and puts your thoughts and mind into complaining mode; let's not quickly forget that complaining is what made the Israelite's relationship with God erode!

Check Point

How often do you entertain thoughts of jealousy? When you do, what are the kinds of things you get jealous about? The Bible says that God is a jealous God (Exodus 34:14), but when God is jealous, He is righteously jealous because He loves us and yearns for us. In the same manner, our healing and health would flourish if we allow only righteous jealousy after God's heart occupy our thoughts and minds.

Exclamation Point !

"Delight yourself also in the Lord, And He shall give you the desires of your heart." – Psalm 37:4

"Affliction brings out graces that cannot be seen in times of health." – R.M. McCheyne

Bonus Word

J can also be for *Juice*; juice is essential to the proper, balanced diet. Juice fasting is a good way to reset your body, and intaking the right amount of juice can help with your fruit intake. Try to avoid concentrated juices, though, as they can be very high in sugar! Having fresh squeezed juice is very helpful, as it turns into sugar 20 minutes after juicing it.

K - Kale

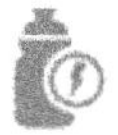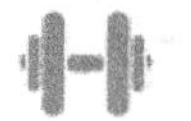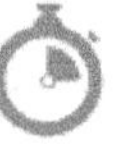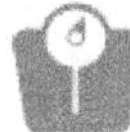

Kale is a superfood that has an acquired taste; there are many ways to prepare it to mask the distinct flavor so that it doesn't go to waste. Adding the right amount of kale to your diet can help your body begin to feel better almost immediately! Eating the right kinds of food is something that we should do obediently.

Health and healing in our bodies depends on the right diet for our specific lifestyle and physical needs; someone who competes in the Olympics would have a higher calorie intake than someone looking to lose weight when they feed. In order to determine your specific dietary needs, seeing a nutritionist is essential; when healthy food is recommended to eat, usually at the top of the list is kale!

It can be baked into crispy chips or tossed in a salad with other greens. It can be added on top of a hamburger instead of lettuce and it's loaded with proteins! It can be added to a smoothie or made into a dip; it aides in better digestion and adds a lot of vitamins and fiber in just one sip!

Check Point

Have you ever tired kale? Why or why not? Out of all the ways mentioned, which one sounds the most appealing to you? Start there when trying it out for the first time!

Exclamation Point

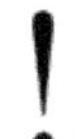

"For as he thinks in his heart, so is he. "Eat and drink!" he says to you, But his heart is not with you." – Proverbs 23:7

Bonus Word 

K can also be for *Kitchen*; having the proper tools and ingredients in your kitchen is essential to health and healing, because not having them can hinder you from having a good meal. An unorganized kitchen can lead to an unorganized diet.

L - Laughter

 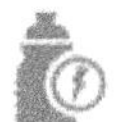 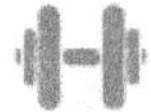 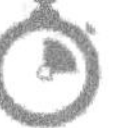  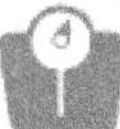

Laughter is one of the best natural medicines out there because it instantly decreases the level of stress hormones your brain releases into your body. A good amount of laughter daily can help you feel less shoddy!

Laughter increases immune cells and infection-fighting antibodies, which means it strengthens your body against disease. Laughter is one of the few natural medicines that can bring instant relief!

Laughter releases endorphins, which are hormones that promote and overall sense of well-being. Laughter is a valuable tool in your journey to health and healing! Doing whatever you can to make sure you laugh as much as possible, especially in situations that would normally be stressful to you, is essential to helping your mind, body, and soul continually pull through!

Check Point

How often do you find yourself laughing? How often do you try to laugh when you are in otherwise stressful circumstances? How could you help yourself loosen up and laugh a little more for the sake of your health and healing?

Exclamation Point !

"And whatever you do in word or deed, do all in the name of the Lord Jesus, giving thanks to God the Father through Him." – Colossians 3:17

"You cannot heal a lifetime of pain overnight. Be patient with yourself; it takes as long as it takes to rebuild yourself." – Anonymous

Bonus Word

L can also be for *Letting Go*; letting go of things that are unhealthy for you and moving on to is essential to your health and healing. Ask yourself today what you need to let go of in order to have a better journey in health and healing!

M - Medicine

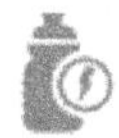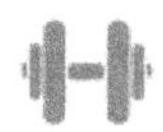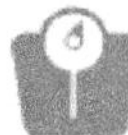

Before there was penicillin, there was God's Word. Before there was ibuprofen, there was God's Word. Before there was chemotherapy and abilities for surgery, there was God's Word. There once was a day when God's Word was the finest medicine ever administered!

Today, God's Word is still the best medicine for any ailment that you may face. God's Word will always provide comfort for you when you're in the middle of your race. God's Word will always heal your soul in places that modern medicine can never touch; God's Word is the best medicine when life feels like it's too much.

Modern medicine has its benefits, too, but God's Word should always be the first medicine we run to. In any situation, God's Word is the medicine that will give us long term health and healing; it's the protection and anointing of God's Word that keeps you healthy in your emotions and feelings!

We can apply the principles of God's Word to our hearts and it will take affect in our minds and bodies over time. If you allow the Holy Spirit to lead you, He will show you new meaning in His Word in the middle of your wartime!

Check Point

When was the last time a doctor prescribed the Word of God to you as medicine? The next time you are facing sickness or health issues, make sure you don't neglect applying the medicine of God's Word!

Exclamation Point !

"Trust in the Lord with all your heart, And lean not on your own understanding; In all your ways acknowledge Him, And He shall direct your paths." – Proverbs 3:5-6

"The words of kindness are more healing to a drooping heart than balm or honey." – Sarah Fielding

Bonus Word 

M can also be for *Memory*; meditating on God's Word, His love for you, praising and worshipping Him, and committing His Word to your memory are all great ways to enhance your journey to health and healing!

N - Nutrition

 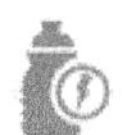 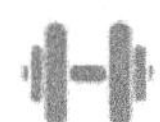 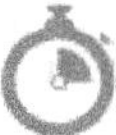  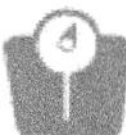

Reading the nutrition labels on every food that you eat is a good habit in your journey to health and healing. Watching your nutrient intake is necessary when rebalancing your diet and how you are feeling.

A lot of the foods sold in grocery stores today contain harmful preservatives and dyes; reading the nutrition label and keeping an eye out for these kinds of things is as essential as exercise!

Being conscience of the nutrition values of food doesn't mean that you can't eat things you like; it means keeping a good balance in what you eat so that your health and blood pressure don't spike!

Nutrition is as simple as being aware of how certain foods affect your body, what value they add to your diet, and what potential problems they might cause.

Nutrition doesn't have to be complicated, but should line up with the Leviticus 23 dietary laws. In Leviticus 23, God gives us insights to what animals He made clean for consumption and which ones would be harmful to our bodies if consumed. Follow these dietary boundaries and principles, and your health and healing will bloom!

Check Point

How often do you pay attention to the nutrition information on the packages of the food you eat? What adjustments would you like to make to your current health habits in order to pay more attention to the nutrition values of your food?

Exclamation Point !

"I beseech you therefore, brethren, by the mercies of God, that you present your bodies a living sacrifice, holy,

acceptable to God, which is *your reasonable service. And do not be conformed to this world, but be transformed by the renewing of your mind, that you may prove what* is *that good and acceptable and perfect will of God."* – Romans 12:1-2

"Healing can be a long and winding road, or a straightforward march to the finish line." – Anonymous

Bonus Word 

N can also be for *Neurogenesis*; neurogenesis is the growth and development of nervous tissue. Science has shown that the human brain is capable of regenerating and healing itself based on repairing negative memories and cells that have been damaged due to emotional and physical trauma. On the road to health and healing, neurogenesis is a noteworthy subject to study!

O — Oral Health

  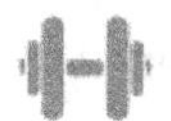   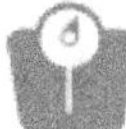

Your mouth is probably the dirtiest, unhealthiest place in the body because it is where the most germs gather. Oral health is essential to overall health and healing, because in the mouth is held the power! Both physically and spiritually speaking, if your mouth is healthy, your body will be healthy, too. Taking good care of your oral health is always the right thing to do!

A mouth that is not properly cared for not only causes pain, but over long periods of time can put your health in serious danger. Infections in the mouth can lead to blood disease, heart failure, and in your own body make you feel like a complete stranger!

Our words also matter when it comes to health and healing, because if we're speaking unhealthy words, it shows what our hearts are truly feeling. Overall, oral health is something that should be paid special attention to when it comes to helping you feel brand new!

Check Point

When is the last time you really paid attention to your oral health? What immediate adjustments would you like to make to start making your mouth both spiritually and physically in better health?

Exclamation Point

"Pray without ceasing, in everything give thanks; for this is the will of God in Christ Jesus for you. Do not quench the Spirit. Do not despise prophecies." – 1 Thessalonians 5:17-20

"Each day comes bearing its own gifts. Untie the ribbons." – Ruth Ann Schabacker

Bonus Word

O can also be for *Oil Pulling*; oil pulling is an ancient health practice where you place a tablespoon of pure coconut oil in your mouth and swish it around for fifteen minutes, then spit it out when done. The oil pulls out bacteria from your gums and helps you maintain a healthy ph. balance in your mouth!

P - Prayer

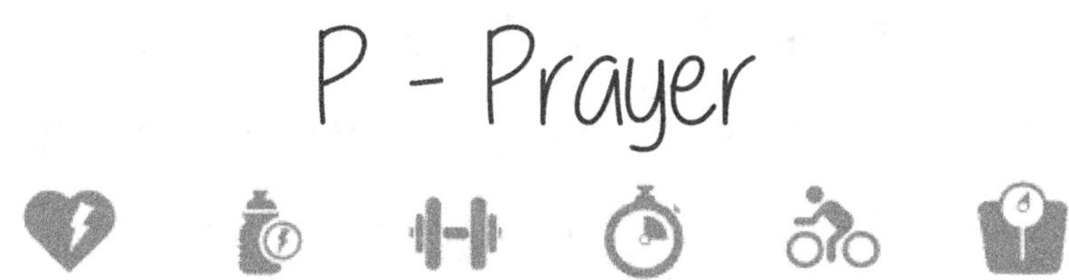

Prayer is one of the most important aspects of health and healing because it is our direct connection and communication with God above. Prayer is our safeguard and open door from heaven, because we obey God out of love.

Prayer releases the kind of anointing from the heavens that is needed for health and healing miracles today. Through the fervent prayer of a righteous person, God brings health and healing our way! The Bible is very clear that it is through prayer that we accomplish health and healing on this earth; it is also through prayer the we confirm to ourselves our heavenly worth!

Prayer should be led by the Holy Spirit and not selfish in nature, but it's also not wrong to pray for the things you need healing in in yourself. If you are sick and in need of healing today, the Bible says you shouldn't sit on a shelf! The Bible says you should go to the elders of the congregation and have them anoint you with oil and pray; the Bible says there is health and healing and forgiveness of sins in this way!

Check Point

When is the last time you prayed about your health and healing? What are some hinderances in your faith that might be keeping you from receiving that health and healing? What are some adjustments you would like to make to your prayer life to become more intimate with God?

Exclamation Point

!

"Rejoice in the Lord always. Again, I will say, rejoice! Let your gentleness be known to all men. The Lord is at

hand. Be anxious for nothing, but in everything by prayer and supplication, with thanksgiving, let your requests be made known to God; and the peace of God, which surpasses all understanding, will guard your hearts and minds through Christ Jesus. Finally, brethren, whatever things are true, whatever things are noble, whatever things are just, whatever things are pure, whatever things are lovely, whatever things are of good report, if there is any virtue and if there is anything praiseworthy—meditate on these things.” – Philippians 4:4-8

“Attitude is a little thing that makes a big difference.” – Winston Churchill

Bonus Word 

P can also be for *Process*; health and healing are a process. They are something that cannot be achieved immediately, but over time through diligent decisions. Don't get discouraged at the process; rejoice in every step along the way!

Q — Questioning Symptoms

 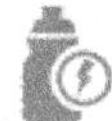 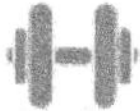 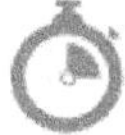 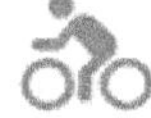 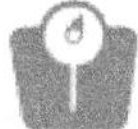

When you are feeling in need of health and healing because you are sick, it's important to question what symptoms you have and what might be causing them. Understanding how you are feeling and what the cause may be can give you a head start on how to address the situation and where it might stem.

Questioning symptoms is also something that should be carefully practiced, because if you go online to figure out what might be ailing you, you might be in for a shock! Some people self-diagnose their symptoms with uneducated guesses from the internet, which can prove to be a crock!

Recording your symptoms and what might have caused them can be a great lead for your doctor to get started in figuring out what's going on; never be afraid to discuss symptoms with your doctor because that is where their research will dawn.

Check Point

When you have a symptom, when do you know to ignore it and when do you know to explore it? Do you currently have any recurring symptoms of any kind? When is the last time you discussed these things with your doctor?

Exclamation Point

!

"Or do you not know that your body is the temple of the Holy Spirit who is in you, whom you have from God, and you are not your own? For you were bought at a price;

therefore glorify God in your body and in your spirit,

which are God's." – 1 Corinthians 6:19-20

"Without faith, God's grace is wasted, and without grace,

faith is powerless." – Andrew Wommack

Bonus Word 

Q can also be for *Quiet Time with God*; having the right
amount of quiet time with God is essential to your health
and healing because it is during these times that we can
clear our mind and hear better from Him.

R - Rest

 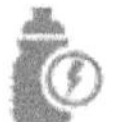 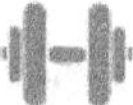 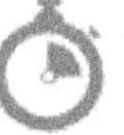  

Rest is essential to health and healing, because without the proper amount of it, you won't even know what you're feeling. A lack of the proper amount of rest can cause anxiety, stress, confusion, and many more things. Insomnia and lack of resting can really grab you where it stings!

Resting is hard sometimes because of the busy lifestyles many lead. However, without resting, your health will deteriorate with incredible speed! Your body does a lot of amazing things while you sleep and rest; new brain cells develop and your body regenerates to operate at its best!

God commanded in the Bible to rest on the Sabbath day and to keep it Holy; to work on six days, but on the seventh day, cease from working fully (Exodus

20:8). God knows what is best for His children, and He commands things for very good reasons. Learning to trust and obey Him is essential in all health and healing seasons!

Check Point

How often do you allow yourself the proper amount of rest? What keeps you from resting the way you need to? What adjustments can you make to your lifestyle to allow yourself more time to rest and recuperate when needed?

Exclamation Point

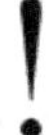

"And whatever you do in word or deed, do all in the name of the Lord Jesus, giving thanks to God the Father through Him." – Colossians 3:17

"Take the first step in faith. You don't have to see the whole staircase, just take the first step." – Dr. Martin Luther King Jr.

Bonus Word 

R can also be for *Reading*; reading the proper materials to know about your body and nutrition is important to health and healing. Reading God's Word daily is also essential to mind health and healing!

S – Scripture

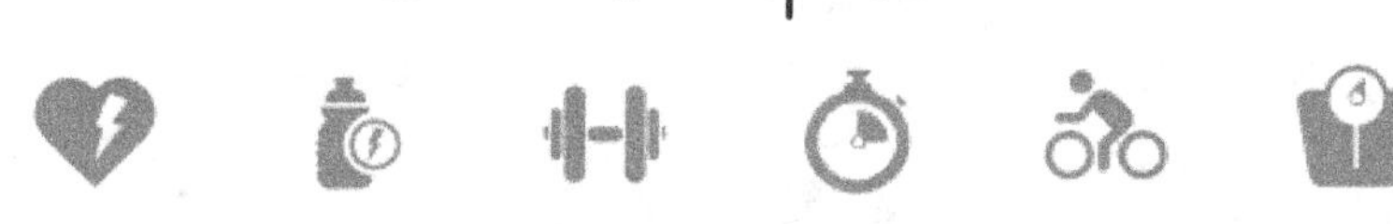

Scripture is God's Word, and it is the finest medicine anyone has seen or heard. Scripture is the all-healing, all-powerful go-to when a believer needs encouragement and vision; the advice and principles in the Scriptures are essential to making healthy, healing decisions!

The amazing thing about the Scriptures is that there are so many things written in there that not only heal our bodies, but our souls and spirits, too. The Scriptures provide health and healing for any situation, physical or spiritual that you could go through!

The Scriptures read in faith, believed upon, spoken aloud and obeyed are the most effective ways of defeating death, hell, and the grave! Without the

Scriptures as our sword and the Holy Spirit inside, health and healing can never abide!

Check Point

How often do you run to God's Word as the first remedy for your sickness in body or soul? What changes can you make in your thought life to put God's Word at the top of the list for remedies to your ailments?

Exclamation Point

!

"This Book of the Law shall not depart from your mouth, but you shall meditate in it day and night, that you may observe to do according to all that is written in it. For then you will make your way prosperous, and then you will have good success. Have I not commanded you? Be strong and of good courage; do not be afraid, nor be

dismayed, for the Lord your God is with you wherever

you go."– Joshua 1:8-9

"You only have so much emotional energy each day.

Don't fight battles that don't matter." – Joel Osteen

Bonus Word 

S can also be for *Sin*; sin can be the main cause and source

of hinderances in health and healing in your life. Ask the

Holy Spirit to reveal in power and might what sin is in

your life that could be hindering your receiving of health

and healing today, then repent and make way for the

healing to come in!

T — Thought Life

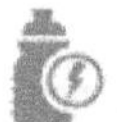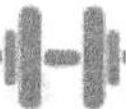

Our thought life is so important to our health and healing, because a sick mind will create a sick body. If you're always thinking about garbage, then your life will be shoddy! Your mind provides the motivation and energy that your body needs to keep going each day; keeping your mind set on negative things will quickly steal your health and healing away!

The Bible teaches many principles on the thought life and how our thoughts should be focused on the things above; if we're always thinking about God and seeking after Him, we will be filled with His love! In the presence of His love, sickness and death cannot abide; when our thought life is filled with His Word, there is nowhere for sickness to hide!

That's not to say that you can simply think yourself into health and healing; but thinking on His thoughts and Words will always change how you are feeling! Instead of despair and discouragement, you'll be filled with peace and hope; a healthy mind will help an unhealthy body not feel like it's at the end of the rope!

Check Point 

How often do you allow your mind to focus on negative things? How do you start to feel after thinking about negative things? What kinds of changes can you make to your thought life to help with your health and healing?

Exclamation Point 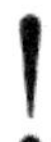

"Let him who is taught the word share in all good things with him who teaches. Do not be deceived, God is not mocked; for whatever a man sows, that he will also reap.

For he who sows to his flesh will of the flesh reap corruption, but he who sows to the Spirit will of the Spirit reap everlasting life. And let us not grow weary while doing good, for in due season we shall reap if we do not lose heart." - Galatians 6:6-9

"Prayer isn't trying to twist God's arm to make Him do something. Prayer is receiving by faith what He has already done!" – Andrew Wommack

Bonus Word 

T can also be for *Taste buds*; your taste buds can sometimes deceive your mind into only wanting a certain flavor of something, or always craving sugar. Don't allow your taste buds to be the one leading you in your diet; you decide what's healthy for you to eat and prepare it in a way that is pleasing to your taste buds!

U - Understanding

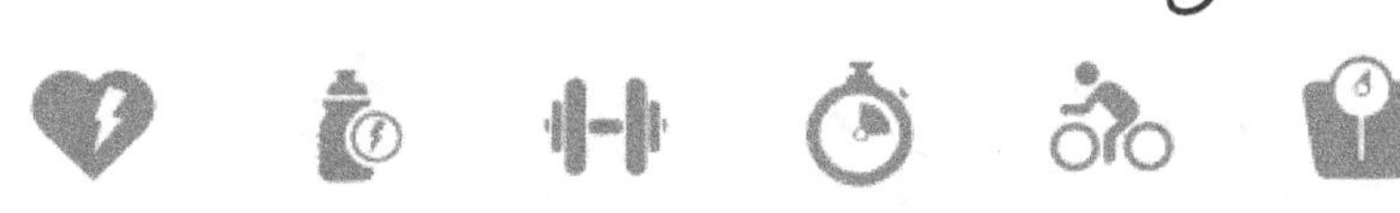

Understanding your body and how it functions will help you keep it healthy. Understanding is always necessary, to every degree. Understanding your own mental health is necessary; understanding how your brain and body works can help you be free!

So often we abuse our bodies on accident simply because we don't understand how it works and what it needs; the same goes for our minds, and on what it feeds. If we train and study and learn about our bodies and minds, we can keep ourselves healthy and avoid sickness of all kinds!

The Bible teaches that gaining understanding is essential and that wisdom is the principle thing. This pertains not only to spiritual matters, but physical matters of health and healing! Understanding your body and how

God designed nature for healing instead of chemicals can help you avoid harmful side effects. Understanding how to harness natural healing remedies is best!

Check Point

How much understanding do you have about how to keep your body healthy, what it needs to survive and thrive, and how to keep it in shape? How about for your mind? What adjustments can you make to gain more understanding in these areas?

Exclamation Point !

"Wisdom is the principal thing;

Therefore get wisdom.

And in all your getting, get understanding.

Exalt her, and she will promote you;

She will bring you honor, when you embrace her.

She will place on your head an ornament of grace;

A crown of glory she will deliver to you."

Hear, my son, and receive my sayings,

And the years of your life will be many.

I have taught you in the way of wisdom;

I have led you in right paths." - Proverbs 4:7-11

"F.A.I.T.H. = Faith Always Is the Healing." - Anonymous

Bonus Word

U can also be for *Underweight*; being underweight is as big a problem as being overweight. If you're one of the many people who struggle with being underweight, it's important to learn how to balance your diet for your metabolism rate. See a nutritionist to help you learn how to increase and enhance your diet to gain the proper amount of weight you need.

V – Vices

  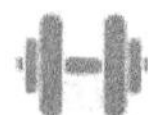 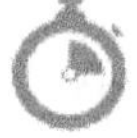  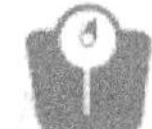

Everyone has vices of some kind; a vice is something that grips you tightly in body and mind. A vice can be like an addiction, only not physically demanding. Sometimes a vice can be as simple as who you lean on most when you need help standing.

Identifying your emotional and physical vices is essential to health and healing; identifying those hidden vices will help you have more power and control over your thoughts and how you're feeling! One of my biggest emotional vices back in the day was pride; I would lean on my own knowledge instead of the Holy Spirit inside.

Take the time to identify your vices today, and ask the Holy Spirit to show you what has to go and what can stay! Don't allow your vices to rule your health in body and mind; evaluate every vice and only keep those whose purpose has been eternally defined!

Check Point

What kind of vices stand in the way of your health and healing in body and mind? Make a list of them and pray over them, submitting them to God and asking Him to give you the power of discernment in which ones must stay and which ones must go.

Exclamation Point

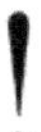

"The grace of the Lord Jesus Christ, and the love of God, and the communion of the Holy Spirit be with you all. Amen." – 2 Corinthians 13:14

"When you hold resentment toward another, you are bound to that person or condition by an emotional link

that is stronger than steel. Forgiveness is the only way to dissolve that link and get free." – Catherine Ponder

Bonus Word 

V can also be for *Verb*; your life is a verb! Your health and healing are a verb! It is something you do, not something you have. Pursue health and healing today, and practice these principles to help you continue in health and healing!

W - Water

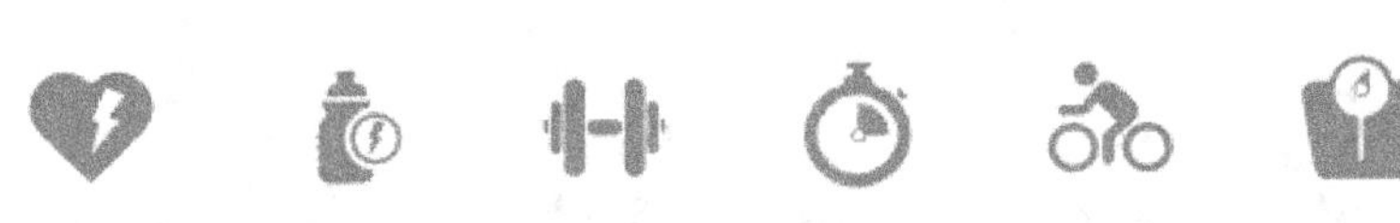

Our bodies consist of between 55-75% of water, which means that hydration is extremely important to our health. Not drinking enough water can cause all kinds of problems, problems that aren't at first obvious, but have stealth.

Dehydration can cause headaches, fatigue, nausea, and more! Not drinking enough water can put you suddenly on the floor! The type of water you drink is also important, because if it is dirty, it will cause more harm than it will good. You must digest water by itself, and not just what is in your food.

Mineral water or alkalized water is essential to health and healing; receiving enough minerals through your water intake can pull out heavy metals from your brain and immediately help how you are feeling!

Check Point

Are you mindful of how much and what type of water you drink? What kinds of adjustments would you like to make to your water intake and why?

Exclamation Point

!

"For Christ did not send me to baptize, but to preach the gospel, not with wisdom of words, lest the cross of Christ should be made of no effect." – 1 Corinthians 1:17

"It is health that is the real wealth, not pieces of gold or silver." – Mahatma Ghandi

Bonus Word

W can also be for *Washing*; washing your hands often is essential to health and healing because germs spread

quickly from hands to mouth. Washing your dishes properly is also essential to health and healing for the same reason. Washing everything properly can keep you healthy and help you avoid contact with germs and diseases!

X - eXcuses

  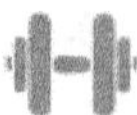 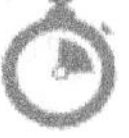  

The more excuses you make, the longer your health and healing will take! Excuses will only keep you from making the needed adjustments to your lifestyle and diet; excuses will only show you what you need for your health and then keep you from trying it!

Excuses are really a disease of the mind; excuses are designed to have you leave your dreams behind! Health and healing won't come as long as you make excuses for why you cannot make changes in your life; making excuses for things will only ever cause strife!

On your journey to health and healing, make sure you ask the Holy Spirit to reveal to you any lingering excuses in your thoughts. Seek and destroy within your mind those lies from the enemy that you have bought!

Check Point 

How many excuses and for how long have you been making excuses when it comes to your health and healing? What do you think would motivate you to finally stop making excuses about your health and healing and pursue it fully?

Exclamation Point !

"And they overcame him by the blood of the Lamb and by the word of their testimony, and they did not love their lives to the death." – Revelation 12:11

"Being deeply loved by someone gives you strength, while loving someone deeply gives you courage." – Lao Tzu

Bonus Word

X can also be for *eXpectations*; having unhealthy expectations will also create in you an unhealthy mindset. Evaluate your expectations today and make sure that they are lining up with God's expectations.

Y — Ylang Ylang

Ylang Ylang essential oil is one of nature's finest antidepressants. Ylang Ylang therapy has been said to make people feel like they are once again in their adolescence!

Inhaling or massage therapy with Ylang Ylang can be very beneficial to your body and soul; ylang ylang is also good for bad skin conditions and can leave you feeling whole! Ylang Ylang helps fight depression and relaxes the body, creating feelings of joy and peace. Ylang Ylang can be effective for emotional therapy as well as physical release!

Health and healing is all about learning the different things God placed in nature to help us with the many things our body may suffer; God knew ahead of

time the challenges of living on this planet and prepared for us several natural buffers!

Check Point

Have you ever tried Ylang Ylang for depression? Why or why not? What was your experience?

Exclamation Point

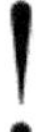

"So then faith comes by hearing, and hearing by the word of God."– Romans 10:17

"With the fearful strain that is on me night and day, if I did not laugh, I should die." – Abraham Lincoln

Bonus Word

Y can also be for *Yawn*; science has previously told us that yawning was a sign that our brain needs more oxygen, but recently, that theory has been disputed. Yawning remains to be one of the few bodily functions that science doesn't fully yet understand!

Z - Zen

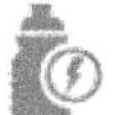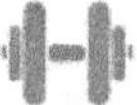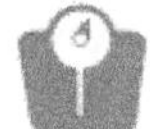

Zen is a word that is used by Buddhists and monks to promote and elevate the importance of meditation and intuition. The Holy Spirit has the only true Zen, which through relationship with Yeshua (Jesus), comes into fruition.

Health and healing depend on the amount of peace and wholeness that you have in your mind, body, and soul. If you ask the Holy Spirit, He will give you His Kingdom, which will make all three of those elements of yourself whole!

The only true Zen in the world comes from meditating on God's Word and relying on the Holy Spirit's direction; nothing about human intuition can promote health and healing or fight off spiritual or physical infection!

Check Point

How often do you meditate on God's Word? How often do you rely on the Holy Spirit's direction for your health and healing? What adjustments do you think should be made to your mediation and reliance on the Holy Spirit and why?

Exclamation Point

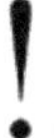

"That if you confess with your mouth the Lord Jesus and believe in your heart that God has raised Him from the dead, you will be saved. For with the heart one believes unto righteousness, and with the mouth confession is made unto salvation. For the Scripture says, "Whoever believes on Him will not be put to shame." For there is no distinction between Jew and Greek, for the same Lord over all is rich to all who call upon Him. For "whoever

calls on the name of the Lord shall be saved."" - Romans 10:9-13

"Our heavenly Father has a thousand ways to provide for us, of which we know nothing." – Ellen G. White

Bonus Word 

Z can also be for *Zeal*; never allow yourself to lose your zeal when it comes to pursuing a lifestyle of health and healing! Ask the Holy Spirit to fill you with zeal all the day long to stay strong!

**For more ABC's titles by
Dr. Chad Costantino,
please visit:**

www.abundantlifepublishing.org